# Acid Reflux Relief

## Relieve your Acid Reflux with 10 Powerful and Safe Natural Remedies

I0482196

# Table of Contents

# Introduction

Hello and welcome to the book all about acid reflux relief. If you have chronic suffering from heartburn, you've come to the right place! Through this book, we will be teaching you about:

- What exactly you are suffering from: Is it heartburn, acid reflux, or GERD?
- What is causing the pain: From physical, to outside factors, to what exactly is happening inside of your body.
- What symptoms you should be aware of.
- What life style changes you can make to help the pain.
- What diet changes you can make to relieve acid reflux.
- Certain foods to consume and avoid in your diet
- Special recipes to help alleviate heartburn
- And more information about heartburn, acid reflux, and GERD

By the end of this book, I hope to make you an acid reflux master. With more than 60 million American adults experiencing heartburn every month, it is probable that you or someone you know suffer from heartburn. Of those 60 million, 15 million suffer daily. If you are one of these individuals, it is time to take steps to help prevent heartburn.

It is important that you realize that many people suffer from this chronic disease. However, this does not mean that you need to sit down and deal with the pain. You should also be aware that sometimes, medicine prescribed by the doctor is not always the best option. More times than not, medication will simply relieve the symptom.

What if you could solve the issue from its very root? We are here to show you that you absolutely can!

Your health is in your own hands. I am here to guide you to a path of healthy living. I will be introducing life style changes including weight loss, stress relievers like aromatherapy, and why elevating your head while you sleep may be a good idea.

I have also included chapters teaching you about what foods are causing your heartburn. In this book, you will find a list of foods to avoid and a list of food that can help sooth your heartburn pains. As if that isn't enough, I have also included simple recipes that can alleviate pain caused by chronic acid reflux.

Now, it is time to begin your acid reflux relief journey. Read the following chapters to learn everything you need to know about the acid reflux and why you may be suffering from the consequences of your life style. By the end, you will be able to help yourself and those who suffer with acid reflux, heartburn and GERD.

The best place to start is the beginning. It is important for you to realize there is a difference between heartburn, acid reflux and GERD. Continue reading to learn more about the causes, symptoms, and factors of each illness. Good luck and we wish you the best on your acid reflux relief journey.

# Chapter One: Understanding Acid Reflux

With more than three million cases per year in the United States, acid reflux is a very common issue with the body. If you have had pains in your chest, it could be a symptom of acid reflux. Before we begin to discuss remedies for the issue, we must first learn what is causing the problems. The body is a complex system that can be altered depending on weight, diet, and family history. If you believe you are suffering from acid reflux, there are several natural steps that can be taken to help relieve these symptoms.

There are several factors that induce reflux. The question is, why is this happening to me? If you have symptoms such as burning in your chest, this may be caused by a valve at the entrance of your stomach called the lower esophageal sphincter, or LES. In a normal situation, the LES will close as soon as food passes through so that stomach acids do not emerge into the esophagus. For some people, the LES does not close all of the way or can sometimes open too often which is when heartburn transpires.

Another common cause of acid reflux is a stomach abnormality known as hiatal hernia. In simple terms, the hernia develops when the LES and the upper part of the stomach migrate above the diaphragm. The diaphragm is a vital piece that separates the stomach from the chest. By doing so, the diaphragm keeps acid where it is supposed to be, in the stomach. If a person develops a hiatal hernia, they are at a higher risk for acid to move into the esophagus, causing acid reflux.

If you are concerned about acid reflux, be aware that more than 60 million Americans experience heartburn at least once a month and about 15 million suffer from daily heartburn. In recent studies, scientists have found that GERD or acid reflux is becoming more common in infants and children, creating respiratory problems from recurrent vomiting and coughing. Pregnant woman can also suffer from daily heartburn due to the body's chemistry.

A pain in the chest region can be a tricky symptom. For some people, this may be simple heartburn while for others, it could be a first symptom of a heart attack. If you experience extreme pain in the chest, a doctor visit is highly suggested. After all, it is better to be safe than sorry. If chest pains are an issue you deal with daily, you may be suffering from heartburn, acid reflux, or GERD. An important fact to realize is that they are not all one in the same. A little case of heartburn is much less serious than GERD. Below, we will explain what each issue is, what factors cause the sickness, and the symptoms of each. This way, you may figure out which one you have and how serious of a problem it can potentially be.

## Heartburn

Heartburn is what most people will call that

burning pain in the chest. Often times, the pain is centered behind the breastbone and can become worse when laying down or bending over. Most people deal with the pain and occasional heartburn. If this is a symptom that occurs every once in a while, there is no need to be alarmed. If the heartburn interferes with your daily routine, the condition may be more severe.

## Symptoms of Heartburn:

- Burning pain in the chest area that mostly occurs after eating or at night time
- The burning pain becomes worse when you are bending over or lying down

## Factors that Cause Heartburn:

While the factors listed below can cause heartburn, being overweight and/or pregnant can increase the risk of experiencing heartburn. If you suffer from pain in your chest, try avoiding the following foods and beverages.

- Alcohol
- Carbonated beverages
- Citrus products (i.e.: Oranges)
- Chocolate
- Fatty meals
- Large meals
- Peppermint
- Spicy food
- Tomato products (i.e.: ketchup)

## Physical Cause of Heartburn:

As stated earlier, the issue that causes heartburn is acid reflux. The heartburn is actually a symptom of the acid reflux which occurs when a person's lower esophageal sphincter is weak or relaxes abnormally. When the stomach acid backs up into the esophagus, this is when the symptoms occur. It will be especially painful if you are laying down or bending over.

If your heartburn occurs more than twice a week, it may be time to go to the doctor. It is important to find out what is going on inside of your body before treating the illness. Some doctors may suggest over-the-counter medication but, this may just help fix the symptoms. Later in the chapters, we will be discussing natural remedies to help cure the acid reflux, not just the symptoms. If you are having problems swallowing, constant vomiting or nausea, or experience weight loss because you are having difficulty eating, a trip to the doctor is necessary.

# **Acid Reflux**

Acid reflux is the chronic disease that happens when stomach acid and bile end up in the esophagus and irritate the lining. If you are experiencing constant heartburn, this may be due to having acid reflux. Constant acid reflux and heartburn could indicate GERD.

## Symptoms of Acid Reflux

- Heartburn is the main symptom of acid reflux. This may be pain or discomfort in your chest, abdomen, or sometimes the throat.
- Burping
- Bloating
- Bloody/black stools
- Bloody vomiting
- Dysphagia- This occurs when the esophagus narrows, which may cause the feeling that there is food stuck in your throat
- Hiccups that will not go away

- Nausea
- Regurgitation- This could mean a sour/ bitter acid that backs up into the throat or mouth
- Wheezing, hoarseness, dry cough, and/or chronic sore throat
- Unexplained weight loss

## Factors that cause Acid Reflux

- Being pregnant
- Being overweight or obese
- Drinking beverages including: alcohol, coffee, carbonated drinks, or tea
- Eating certain foods including: citrus, chocolate, garlic, fatty foods, onions, spicy foods, or tomatoes
- Eating heavy meals
- Eating large meals
- Eating while laying down or bending over
- Smoking
- Snacking close to bed time
- Taking medications such as aspirin, blood pressure medications, ibuprofen, or certain muscle relaxers

## Diagnosis of Acid Reflux

Seeing that I have already discussed what physically causes acid reflux, you should be aware if you have the symptoms. If you feel you are suffering from acid reflux, it is time to visit your doctor for a professional's view. While at the doctor, there are several tests that can be used to diagnose acid reflux.

- **Barium Swallow**- Also known as an esophagram, this procedure checks to see if your esophagus narrows or if there are any ulcers. During the test, you will be swallowing a solution in which can show any abnormalities in an x-ray.

- **Biopsy**- This can be taken during an endoscopy to check the sample tissue for any infection or abnormalities within the body.
- **Endoscopy**- The endoscopy test checks to see if there are any problems in the esophagus or the stomach. During the procedure, a doctor will first spray the back of your throat with an anesthetic and/or a sedative so that you will be comfortable. Next, they will insert a long, lighted tube down the throat to get a look of what is going on inside of your body.
- **Esophageal Manometry**- This procedure helps check the function of your lower esophageal sphincter and your esophagus. This is done by measuring the rhythmic muscle contractions your esophagus makes when you swallow with a thin catheter that is passed through the nose. An esophageal manometry also measures the coordination and force the esophagus makes when passing food.
- **pH monitoring**- The pH monitoring procedure is done by a doctor who inserts a device into the esophagus that stays in place for one to two days. This is done to measure the amount of acid in the esophagus. If the acid level is higher than normal, acid reflux may be the culprit and steps can be taken to help lower the acidity in the body.

# GERD

GERD stands for Gastroesophageal Reflux Disease. This is the issue behind constant acid reflux and the symptom of heartburn. GERD occurs when the esophageal sphincter is compromised, causing acid to come into the esophagus. This condition can sometimes be caused by hiatal hernias, which I described earlier in the chapter. Luckily, GERD can be relieved through a diet and lifestyle change which we will be learning about later. Although some doctors may offer medication, these medications often will only treat the symptoms. I will be offering safe, natural remedies to get your life back on track and pain free.

For those that do have hiatal hernias, this may be what is weakening the LES. As described earlier, hiatal hernias develop when the upper part of the stomach ends up in the chest and through the small opening of the diaphragm. Due to the fact that the diaphragm is the muscle that separates the abdomen from the chest, this is when people experience acid reflux as they have a higher risk of getting stomach acid into the esophagus.

## Symptoms of GERD

- Heartburn is the most common symptom of GERD. This can also be called acid indigestion
- A sensation of food coming back into the mouth, tasting like acid

## Factors that Cause GERD

- Alcohol
- Chocolate
- Coffee
- Fried/ fatty foods
- Obesity
- Peppermint
- Pregnancy
- Smoking

On top of dietary and life style causes, there are also several medications that have been linked to causing GERD through ways of interfering with the digestive process, relaxing the LES, or irritating the esophagus that may already be inflamed. These medications include:

- Some antibiotics
- Anticholinergics
- Some asthma medications i.e.: Albuterol
- Bisphosphonates
- Calcium channel blockers
- Iron tablets
- Non-steroidal anti-inflammatory drugs (NSAIDs)
- Painkillers
- Potassium
- Sedatives

Although these medications can cause issues with the upper digestive track, never stop taking medication without consulting your doctor. If you feel you are on a medication that is causing heartburn, talk to a professional to see if there is a different medication or a lower dosage to help the pain. You should never take it upon yourself to fix the issue.

## Physical Cause of GERD

People of all ages can develop hiatal hernias. Some studies have found that many healthy people over the age of 50 often times have a small hiatal hernia. Doctors believe that the hiatal hernias can be caused by coughing, straining, vomiting or sudden physical exertion. These actions sometimes cause pressure within the abdomen and create a hiatal hernia.

Due to the fact the hernias are somewhat common, they usually do not require treatment. However, sometimes a hernia has the potential to become dangerous if they were to become strangulated. This meaning that the hernia can twist and cut off blood supply, causing a paraesophageal hernia. The hernia may also be complicated by esophagitis and in turn, may need a doctor to reduce the size of the hernia through surgery.

By being aware of your symptoms, you should be aware if it is time to go see a professional or not. While preparing for a doctor visit, there a few preliminary steps that can be taken to make the process a bit easier. You should make a list including:

- **Medications**- This can include vitamins or supplements you may be taking.
- **Medical information**- Discuss with your doctor what conditions you have. In some cases, some medical conditions may be leading to your heartburn.
- **Personal information**- Your doctor may ask you if there has been any recent changes or stressors in your life. If there have been big changes such as financial stressors, a recent death, or relationship problems, they could all be contributing to your heartburn and acid reflux.
- **Pre-appointment restrictions**- If you make an appointment, be sure to be aware if you have any restrictions. An example of this is not eating solid foods 24 hours before your appointment.
- **Symptoms**– Writing down your symptoms is incredibly important. If you are experiencing heartburn, vomiting, or weight loss, tell your doctor everything that is happening. You should report any symptom, even if it seems unrelated to the issue.
- **Questions**- Before attending an appointment with your doctor, you should do some research about what you feel your condition may be and ask the doctor questions you may be concerned about. Try questions such as:
  1. Can I treat myself or do I need medication?
  2. What foods can make my heartburn worse?
  3. Can losing weight help the symptoms?

4. How do I know if the problem is more serious?
5. What treatments are available to treat my issue?
6. Am I on any medications that may be causing heartburn?
7. Do I have any medical conditions causing the pain?
8. What symptoms should I be looking for?
9. What lifestyle changes can I make to help heartburn?
10. How will my life be affected by heartburn, acid reflux or GERD in the long run?

# Chapter Two: Safe and Natural Remedies for Acid Reflux

Now that you are aware of the differences between heartburn, acid reflux, and GERD, it is time to learn how to treat the pain. I want to introduce natural remedies for the illness because sometimes, drugs have side effects that can make you feel worse, or it may be drugs that are causing the pain in the first place!

Common medications that can cause heartburn include antibiotics, antidepressants, anxiety medications, blood pressure medication, nitroglycerin, osteoporosis medication, and even pain relievers. These certain medications can inhibit pain through a number of reasons. One way to avoid pain is by taking the recommended dosage. If you take more than prescribed, heartburn can occur. Sometimes, the fix is as simple as taking medication on an empty stomach. Be sure that when your doctor or pharmacist assigns a medication, you check the directions. If the dosage seems too high, ask your doctor to change the dose or switch to another medication to help heartburn.

A common issue with treating acid reflux with medication is that many people believe acid reflux is caused by an excessive amount of acid in the stomach. Often times, acid-blocking drugs are recommended to help treat the problem. On contrary, the problem is usually a result from having too little acid in the stomach.

There are approximately over 16,000 medical articles showing that stomach acid suppressers do not fix the problem. Instead, they temporarily treat the symptoms. When a doctor prescribes proton pump inhibitors (PPIs), they are effective with blocking the acid production in the body, but this is not a long term solution. PPIs have also been known to have severe side effects such as bone loss, hip fractures, and pneumonia.

Another downfall of being prescribed proton pump inhibitors such as Nexium or Prilosec is that some people have developed a dependence of the drug. In most cases, users will need to wean themselves off of the drug so that they do not experience a rebound of the symptoms they were initially trying to treat. If you were to cut cold turkey, the issue may end up coming back worse than before.

Instead of becoming dependent upon drugs, perhaps it is time to try some natural remedies and a life style change. In this book, I am offering free life style changes you can make yourself and natural remedies that can help treat your illness in a safe way. You do not need to suffer any longer from GERD, acid reflux or the nasty heartburn that comes with them. Continue reading to learn how you can lay your pain to rest.

## 10 Natural Remedies for Acid Reflux

1. **Maintain a healthy weight**
   As stated earlier, obesity can contribute to acid reflux. The excess pounds on the body can place pressure onto the abdomen and in return, press onto the stomach where the acid can back up into the esophagus. Losing weight is one of the most effective ways to relieve your acid reflux symptoms. People usually start noticing improvements after losing just a few pounds!
2. **Wear comfortable clothing**
   Current trends include tight clothes. These styles may be pressing onto the abdomen and the lower esophageal sphincter, forcing acid into the esophagus. By wearing comfortable or looser fitting clothing, this problem can be avoided all together.
3. **Quit Smoking**
   Smoking can decrease the lower esophageal

sphincter's ability to function efficiently. If this happens, the acid will rise into the esophagus and cause heartburn. Smoking also increases acid secretion and it damages the esophageal lining. People who smoke also have less saliva production. Saliva contains bicarbonate which neutralizes acid and helps to minimize damage to your esophagus. Reduced saliva can take away some of your protection. Most of us are already aware of how bad smoking is for not only us, but for the people around us. Do yourself a favor and quit the habit to perhaps stop your pain.

4. **Avoid trigger foods**

In the next chapter, I will be giving you a list of foods to eat and a list of foods to avoid while trying to subdue your heartburn. If you look at the foods listed, you may find the culprit of your pain.

5. **Do not lay down after a meal**

For some people, the issue behind their heartburn and acid reflux may be a simple fix. It is suggested that people wait a minimum of three hours before laying down. If the body is in a parallel position, this may increase the risk of stomach acid coming up into the esophagus.

6. **Avoid eating late**

Obviously if the chances of heartburn are increased when laying down or bending over, you will want to avoid eating just before bed time. Instead, try eating an earlier dinner so your food has a chance to digest and settle before going to sleep.

7. **Elevating head levels**

If you have tried avoiding eating late and laying down after a meal and are still experiencing heartburn at night, it may be time to elevate your head level. Lying flat keeps your throat and stomach at the same level which makes it easier for acids to flow up your esophagus. Most times, elevating the head with an additional pillow is not efficient enough. There are specially designed wedge pillows that should be used instead. These wedge pillows can be purchased online. You can also try inserting a wedge in between your mattress and box spring to help elevate the body from the waist.

8. **Try Melatonin**

    Melatonin is a supplement that is known to help benefit sleep. However, it is increasingly being used to treat acid reflux. Melatonin can lower gastric acid secretion as well as control the lower esophageal sphincter which allows it to close more effectively. While melatonin is a natural supplement, you should still consult with your doctor before taking it.

9. **Quit the processed foods**

    If your diet consists of mostly processed foods and sugar, the issue may be in the bacterial balance in your stomach. Instead of filling yourself with foods that are processed, try eating natural foods that are high-quality, organic, and natural. I will list foods that will help sooth heartburn in a later chapter.

10. **Sit back and Relax**

    One of the biggest culprits that cause heartburn symptoms are anxiety and stress. If you experience heightened pain when you are stressed out, there are a few methods to consider to help painful symptoms.

    - Aromatherapy
    - Exercise- Try gentle exercises such as walking or riding a bike. If exercise is too vigorous, this may increase the pain.
    - Hypnosis
    - Massage
    - Music- Try a gentle genre or nature sounds to help relax

# Chapter Three: Food List for Acid Reflux Relief

Before I begin discussing the list of foods to avoid and consume for acid reflux relief, readers should first be aware of their portion sizes. I have already discussed cutting out processed foods to help relieve symptoms but eating healthy is not equivalent to eating in excess portions. By decreasing portion sizes during meal time, this may help relieve acid reflux symptoms. Decreased portion sizes can also lead to weight loss which can help alleviate the painful symptoms of acid reflux.

## Foods to Avoid

- **Beverages-** Try your best to avoid beverages including coffee, liquor, tea, and wine. Beverages including alcohol relax the LES, causing your heartburn. Other times, a glass of wine may not lead to heartburn, but if you are drinking the glass of wine with a particularly citrusy or fatty meal, it may cause an overload on your body.
- **Chocolate-** This can cause heartburn for a couple of different reasons. First, chocolate can have caffeine that causes heartburn. However, chocolate also relaxes the LES the same as alcohol can, giving the ability for acid to rise into the esophagus. Basically, you want to avoid foods that cause the LES to relax, especially if yours does not function properly beforehand.
- **Dairy-** If you are experiencing heartburn, dairy may be the cause. There is a misconception that milk can relieve heartburn but it is very temporary. The milk acts as a buffer for stomach acid but then can stimulate the stomach to produce more acid. It is best to avoid dairy products such as whole milk, sour cream, ice cream, and cottage cheese. If you do

want to have milk, stick with skim milk and keep your portions small.

- **Fruits and Fruit Juices-** These can include items such as: Cranberry, grapefruit, lemon, and orange. Try to avoid the juices that come from the fruit as well. These fruits are bad for our system because they are so acidic. If these fruits are consumed on an empty stomach, they are more likely to cause heartburn.
- **Fats, Oils, and Sugar-** Foods that include fats, oils, and sugar is very bad for your health. One should try their best to avoid fried and fatty foods in their diet. These foods include potato chips, oily salad dressings, and sweets such as brownies, cookies, and doughnuts. Other foods that are high in fat that you should avoid include avocadoes, cheese, and nuts. Fat slows the stomach down from becoming empty and in return, creates a higher risk of getting a distended stomach. If the stomach becomes enlarged, this increases the pressure on the esophageal sphincter, causing heartburn.
- **Garlic-** Garlic has been known to cause heartburn. According to doctors, this is an individual issue. While some people have no issue with garlic, others who are more prone to heartburn should avoid garlic and onions.
- **Grains-** Some grains may cause heartburn. Try avoiding foods such as spaghetti and macaroni and cheese.
- **Meats-** As for meat, try to avoid chicken wings, chicken nuggets, ground beef and sirloin.
- **Peppermint-** The same as dairy, there is a misconception that peppermint can soothe the stomach. If you are prone to heartburn, avoid peppermint the best you can. Peppermint causes the sphincter muscle to relax which is bad if you want the muscle to function properly and stop

stomach acid from flowing into the esophagus. While the mint may be great for your date, think of your body before popping a mint into your mouth.

- **Spicy Foods-** Foods including chili and Mexican foods are often filled with spices that trigger heartburn. If you feel your symptoms become worse after consuming spicy foods, try to cut it out of your diet. If anything, eat the food in smaller portions so there is a slimmer chance of experiencing the symptoms.
- **Tomatoes-** With the same concept as the citrus fruits, tomatoes are very acidic. Although tomatoes have many health benefits, they may also cause heartburn. Try avoiding ingredients that include tomatoes such as ketchup and pasta sauce.

## Foods to Help Acid Reflux

- **Bread-** When choosing breads, avoid the ones that have been stripped of their natural nutrients, fiber, and vitamins. Find whole-grain bread to help avoid heartburn symptoms of acid reflux.
- **Dessert-** Of course, you will not want to cut out dessert from your diet. You are already suffering from heartburn, why increase the mental pain of having to cut off dessert? You can have dessert in moderation. Try desserts such as angel food cake, low-fat cookies and ice cream, frozen yogurt, sherbet, sponge cake, and hard candy.
- **Egg whites-** If you want eggs in your diet, skip the yolk. You will want to consume the egg whites because they are low in acid.
- **Fish-** Having fresh fish can be great for any diet. It is recommended you look for wild fish as opposed to farm-raised ones. When cooking, try baked, grilled or poached. If you suffer from acid reflux,

you will want to avoid frying fish and using fatty sauces. As for other seafood, try lobster, shrimp and shellfish to include in your diet.

- **Fruits-** You will want to stick with fruits that are low in acid content. Try fruits such as bananas, cantaloupe, honeydew, melons, and watermelon. These foods are great to have as snacks or include in certain meals.
- **Ginger-** Ginger is known as one of the best foods to fight acid reflux and has been used for generations. Ginger is great to use for cooking or adding into smoothies.
- **Healthy fats-** Fats can be hard to avoid in a diet. Instead, try sticking with healthy fats including nuts, seeds, low-fat mayonnaise and salad dressings. While cooking, try using small amounts of olive, vegetable, and sunflower oil.
- **Lean meats and poultry-** As you learned earlier, fatty foods and meats are bad for your system and increase the chances of experiencing heartburn. Try sticking with lean meats such as chicken and turkey. Avoid frying these foods at all cost. Instead, bake, grill, broil, or steam the meat. In moderation, ground beef and steak can be fine to include in your diet. If pain persists, cut the two from your diet all together.
- **Oatmeal-** Oatmeal is full of healthy fiber and a great way to start the day! Its natural grains are low in acid and will not cause reflux.
- **Potatoes-** When it comes to consuming vegetables, stick with root vegetables such as ginger, parsnips, radish, carrots and potatoes. These vegetables are rich in nutrients and low in acid.
- **Rice-** Look for rice such as brown rice because it is high in fiber. Complex carbs are great to include in

the diet in order to combat reflux symptoms. Couscous can also be another diet alternative to processed white rice.

- **Vegetables-** There are some vegetables that are low in acid and will not cause heartburn. Look for vegetables including: asparagus, broccoli, celery, cauliflower and green beans.

## Beverages for Acid Reflux Relief

- **Herbal Tea-** Tea can be a great beverage to help soothe stomach issues and improve digestion in some cases. Most caffeine-free herbal teas are fine to have minus spearmint or peppermint. The teas recommended for digestion include chamomile, licorice, marshmallow, and slippery elm. For best results, one should drink two to four cups of this tea per day.
- **Non-Citrus Juice-** As we learned earlier, acidic fruits are bad for our system and should be avoided at all cost. Stay away from fruit juices such as grapefruit, orange, and pineapple. Instead, try fruit juices from apples, Aloe Vera, cabbage, and carrot.
- **Skim Milk-** If you want to include a milk in your diet, try skim or goat's milk. Unfortunately, regular whole milk contains a lot of fat and can worsen reflux symptoms. If possible, only drink 8 ounces of skim milk. You want to avoid overfilling the stomach as it may increase the chances of heartburn by overextending the stomach.
- **Water-** Water should be a normal art of your diet. As recommended, you should be getting at least eight glasses of water a day. Some doctors will suggest drinking alkaline water to help control acid reflux and reduce stomach acidity.

# Chapter Four: Acid Reflux Relief Recipes

Now that we are aware of what foods to avoid and which foods to include in the diet, I have decided to include a few recipes to get you started on the road to acid reflux relief. The following recipes include all food to help soothe acid reflux symptoms and can be used for all meals of the day. There are many resources including acid reflux relief recipes to keep your diet fresh and exciting.

**Smoothie**

**Almond Milk Smoothie**
*Servings: 2*

Ingredients:

- ½ cup of Greek yogurt
- 6 strawberries
- ½ cup of pineapple
- 1 teaspoon of turmeric
- 1 cup of almond milk
- 1 cup of apple juice

Directions:

Place all of the ingredients into a blender and blend until smooth.

**Breakfast**

**Muesli Oatmeal**
*Servings: 2*

Ingredients:

- 1 cup of instant oatmeal
- ½ banana
- ½ apple

- 2 teaspoons of honey
- 2 tablespoons of raisins
- 1 cup of skim milk
- Optional: Salt

Directions:

1. The night before you plan on eating your meal, mix the oatmeal, skim milk, raisins, and honey into a bowl.
2. Next, cover the mixture and place into your refrigerator.
3. The next morning, check the consistency. If it is too thick, try adding milk.
4. Last, add fruit to the mixture and your meal is ready to eat!

## Lunch

### Mushroom Quesadilla

*Servings: 4*

Ingredients:

- 4 whole wheat flour tortillas
- 4 Portobello mushroom caps
- 4 cups of baby spinach
- 1 cucumber
- 1 avocado
- 4 ounces of Swiss cheese
- ½ cup of fresh cilantro
- 2 tablespoons of olive oil
- 2 tablespoons of rice wine vinegar
- Low fat sour cream
- Optional: Pepper

## Directions:

1. Heat a pan over the oven on medium heat.
2. In a separate bowl, mix your avocado and cucumber with the vinegar and one tablespoon of oil. Once these are mixed together, add the ½ cup of fresh cilantro.
3. On a baking sheet, place your whole wheat tortillas and sprinkle cheese on half. Once cheese is placed, top the same half with the baby spinach.
4. Place the mushrooms into the pan and cover with the rest of the olive oil. Grill these for about 3 to 4 minutes on both sides.
5. When mushrooms are cooked, place on top of the spinach and close the tortillas. Grill the folded tortillas for about 2 minutes for each side.
6. If desired, serve tortillas with a side of cucumber, avocado and a dollop of sour cream.

## Dinner

### Spinach Lasagna
*Servings: 4*

## Ingredients:

- 1 10-ounce package of spinach
- 1 12-ounce package of winter squash puree
- 4 ounces of non-fat Mozzarella cheese
- 15 ounces of Lite Ricotta cheese
- ½ cup of grated Parmesan cheese
- 6 oven ready lasagna noodles
- ¼ teaspoon of pepper
- 1/8 teaspoon of ground nutmeg
- 1/8 teaspoon of turmeric

## Directions:

1. Begin by pre-heating your oven to 425 degrees.
2. In a bowl, combine your cheeses with the seasonings. Once these are mixed together, you will want to add the spinach to it.
3. In a square pan, begin to spread ½ cup of the winter squash puree in the bottom.
4. Once this is done, top the squash with two of the noodles and spread 1/3 of the squash over the top of those.
5. When this has been finished, place 1/3 of the spinach and cheese mixture on top.
6. Add two more of the noodles on top of the mixture and add another 1/3 of the squash.
7. You should cover the lasagna with a piece of foil that has been lightly oiled and proceed by baking for about 15 minutes.
8. After time has been allotted, uncover the lasagna and bake for another ten minutes. The top should be a nice, golden brown color.

## Dessert

### Banana Sorbet
*Servings: 4*

<u>Ingredients:</u>

- 3 bananas
- 2 tablespoons of honey
- 1 tablespoon of ginger
- 1/8 teaspoon of ground cardamom
- 3 cups of ice
- ¼ teaspoon of salt.

<u>Directions:</u>

1. In a blender, place the bananas, honey, ginger, cardamom, and salt and blend on high.
2. Once this is done, add the ice until sorbet has

reached a consistency desired.
3. This recipe can be served immediately or stored in freezer for dessert later.

# Conclusion

At this point in the book, you should be an acid reflux expert. Just to recap, you have learned:

- The differences between heartburn, acid reflux, and GERD
- The symptoms and factors
- 10 natural remedies for acid reflux
- Foods to consume and avoid if you suffer from GERD
- Acid reflux friendly recipes to get started

If you, or someone you know suffers from heartburn, acid reflux, or GERD, you now realize that suffering is no longer permitted. If you feel you may have one of these issues, it is time to get checked out by a doctor. If they tell you that you have acid reflux or GERD and try to assign you medication, you can feel free to try to treat it yourself.

By following our natural remedies, life style changes, food lists, and recipes, you should begin to see a difference in your health. A scary part of pain can be from not knowing what is causing it. Now you know that it is the LES causing your pain that is allowing stomach acid to come back into the esophagus. Take the pre-cautions with your diet to help sooth your heartburn.

If you make the diet changes and still experience chronic pain, you may need the medication but remember, medication may be only treating the symptoms. If you feel you need to be prescribed medicine, do so but also change your life style to help lead a pain-free life. There is no harm in being healthy. I wish you the best of luck with your condition and hope my tips have made your life a little easier and a little more pain free.

Thank you so much for purchasing my book! If you received value from it I would be grateful if you would leave a review.


Best Wishes,


Michael

www.ingramcontent.com/pod-product-compliance
Lightning Source LLC
Chambersburg PA
CBHW070429190526
45169CB00003B/1472